EATING SWEET BUT VEGAN

Lauren Webber

Copyright © 2022 by Lauren Webber

All rights reserved.

No portion of this book may be reproduced in any form without written permission from the publisher or author, except as permitted by U.S. copyright law.

Contents

Chapter One

Introduction

I'm happy that you are ready to learn more about the world of delicious, and good-for-you desserts, according to a vegan. You will find many recipes in this book that will help you bring together vegan recipes and healthy habits. They will also help you and those you care about reach a satisfying and nutritious end to your meals.

You should be motivated to become a vegan because it is a very smart decision. With delicious desserts, you will be glad to eat them every day.

A balanced vegan diet has been shown to produce healthy weight loss and lower BMI. Vegetarians of all diets fall within the normal range of BMI, and vegans are the skinniest population in the United States. In fact, the amount of meat one eats is more important in body weight than other dietary issues, such as whether one uses dairy products or not.

Contrary to what our friends and relatives may believe, vegans aren't strict eaters. Instead, they enjoy the natural taste of vegan desserts more than any dessert they have ever eaten. In addition, they become healthier and stronger. Finally, the act of sharing a dessert in a non-violent way helps people to reduce their tension at workplace, school, etc.

In this amazing book will find amazing desserts recipes, and those desserts were created with the help of friends from the vegan community. The list of the desserts recipes I wrote, with the assistance of friends, is to show that there are many original ways to create delicious recipes, which do not harm any animals.

Before we start, I want to show my appreciation for your support in making "101 healthy vegan burgers" a success. It was a pleasure for me to work with you to make this cookbook become a reality. It is my opinion that together, we can make a difference in the world. Also, I want to once again thank you for purchasing "101 healthy vegan burgers", and I wish you all a wonderful learning experience.

Chapter Two

Vegan Cakes

I have to admit that I've been addicted to cakes for a while now. But because of the lack of vegan cakes, I've never taken off the mask of a vegan. When I decided to eventually become a vegan, I realized that I had to take responsibility for my sweet appetite and find vegan cake recipes. It's surprising to find out that vegan cakes can be equally successful. In this chapter, you will find several impressive and tasty cakes, as well as a few for beginners.

Coconut Cake with Chocolate Ganache This moist cake is coated with chocolate ganache. Make sure to serve it on a cake stand so you can admire the lovely shape and color.

Servings: 4-6 dishes

Ingredients:

Cake:

1 cup sugar

4 tablespoons ground flax seeds

8 tablespoons water

3/4 cup coconut flour

1/2 cup all purpose flour,

[2/3 cup of cocoa powder]

1 teaspoon baking powder

1/2 teaspoon baking soda

Use 1 1/4 cup of coconut milk

1 teaspoon vanilla extract

1 pinch of salt

Dark chocolate ganache:

I want to enjoy dark chocolate

4 oz coconut cream

1 tablespoon almond butter

Directions:

Mix the ground flax seeds with water. Make sure they soak for at least 5-10 minutes.

Add the butter and sugar into the bowl and beat them until they are light and fluffy. Add the crushed seeds and the vanilla extract and mix them all together.

3.

Starting with a bit of flour, gradually add in a bit of butter with the milk. At the end of this, mix for a couple of minutes.

5. In an all-butter dish, mix and pour the ingredients. Bake at 350F for 30-40 minutes.

After all this, the recipe said, to make the ganache, I added the coconut cream to the chopped chocolate. Then I thoroughly combined the mixture, added the butter, and poured the ganache over the cake.

Orange Cranberry Cake

The cake is a perfect breakfast in the morning, next to a cup of tea or a glass of warm milk. With just a few ingredients and a small amount of effort, you can prepare this for yourself.

Servings: 4-6 dishes

Ingredients:

¼ cup all purpose flour.

1 tbs baking powder

Orange zest is a great way to add flavor and nutrition to a dish.

1 cup sugar

1 cup of coconut milk

1 cup cooked cranberries.

1 pinch of salt

Directions:

1. In a bowl, mix the salt with the sugar, milk, and orange zest.

3. Sift together the flour, baking powder and salt, add the cranberries, egg, butter and milk.

4. Pour this batter into a small greased cake pan.

1. Heat on 350° F for 30 minutes or until fragrant.

Marbled Banana Bread

The recipe for banana bread includes bananas, oil, buttermilk, eggs, vanilla, honey, and other ingredients. You can also include chocolate chips or coconut flakes and make a delicious new treat.

Servings: 4-6 dishes

Ingredients:

1/2 cup mashed bananas

1/2 Cup Brown Sugar

A cup of vanilla

3 tablespoons vegetable oil

Use 1/3 cup soy milk

1/4 cup whole wheat flour

1 teaspoon baking soda

Baking powder.

4 tablespoons cocoa powder

6 teaspoons of hot water

1 pinch of salt

Directions:

1. Grease or lightly oil the pan and set aside.

Pour the bananas in a bowl, add sugar, vanilla, oil, and soy milk. Stir until blended.

Add flour, baking soda and powder, and salt in a different bowl.

Combine the ingredients in a bowl. Mix them well.

While one part of the batter remains as it is, in the other part, water is added to the same amount of cocoa powder.

6. Pour the batter into the prepared pan, one at a time. Now marble the mixture with a skewer.

Bake in a preheated oven at 350 for 30-40 minutes.

Heat up your leftovers and serve with a sprinkle or powdered sugar.

Chocolate Mint Cake

Chocolate cake is an old-fashioned classic, but add a little twist by dropping some mint on top and you have a real treat!

Servings: 4-6 dishes

Ingredients:

I/4 cup olive oil

1/4 cup melted chocolate

1/4 cup sugar

1 tablespoon flax seeds, ground

2 tablespoons water

1/2 cup flour

1 tablespoon of mint extract

1/2 teaspoon baking powder

⅛

Directions:

Flax seeds can be soaked in water for 10 minutes.

2. Combine the sugar with the oil and melted chocolate. Add the flour and baking powder, followed be the mint extract and a pinch of salt.

3. Grease a small baking pan with oil.

4. Cook in a preheated oven at 350F for about 30-40 minutes.

This cake is the perfect way to celebrate yourself.

Red wine and chocolate make a delicious combination, and this cake is moist and flavorful.

Servings: 4-6 dishes

Ingredients:

3 tablespoons flax seeds, ground

6 tablespoons water

1/2 cup (or less) brown sugar

6 tablespoons olive oil

½ cup red wine

1 teaspoon of vanilla

1 cup of all purpose flour

2 tablespoons chocolate powder

1/2 teaspoon cinnamon

1 teaspoon baking powder.

1 pinch of salt

Directions:

1. You need to soak your flax seeds for five minutes to get the right consistency.

3. Put the oil and sugar together and mix well.

3.

Mix

Incorporate the dry ingredients into the oil mixture. (use different order: oil mixture, then dry)

Spread the batter in a 9-inch round pan.

5. Use this recipe for brownies. Use this recipe for brownies.

Coconut and Orange Cake

This cake tastes like sunshine. It is tropical and moist and you will love it. If you don't like coconut, don't worry. You will love it.

Servings: 4-6 dishes

Ingredients:

1/2 cup coconut flour

4 tablespoons flax seeds, ground

8 tablespoons water

4th of a cup of coconut milk

1/4 cup coconut oil

1/2 cup brown sugar

1 1/2 teaspoon orange zest

2 pinch of salt

1 teaspoon baking powder

4 tablespoons orange juice

1 pinch of salt

Directions:

Mix the flax meal into lukewarm water. Set aside for 5 minutes. 2. After waiting the recommended period, stir the flax into your favorite snack or breakfast cereal. Par

Add the sugar, vanilla, orange zest and juice and mix. Then slowly mix in the coconut oil, melted and chilled. Then add the coconut flour, baking powder and baking soda, and a pinch of salt.

3. Pour a cake mix into a greased and floured pie pan. Bake in a preheated oven at 350F for 50 minutes. Remove from oven and let cool, then sprinkle with powdered sugar. Serve sliced as shown.

Applesauce Spice Cake

Applesauce is very nutritious and gives your cake a moist and fruity flavor. Loaded with autumn flavors, it will flood your house with sweet scents.

Servings: 4-6 dishes

Ingredients:

2 cups all-purpose flour

3/4 cup sugar

1 teaspoon baking soda

1/2 teaspoon baking powder

1 teaspoon cinnamon

1 teaspoon ground ginger.(Paraphrased and added a bold title for emphasis

1/3 cup golden raisins

1/2 cup of chopped walnuts

1 tablespoon, olive oil

11/2 cup of applesauce”

1/2 teaspoon of salt

One teaspoon of vanilla extract

Directions:

1. In a bowl, mix the flour, sugar, baking powder and salt; as well as the cinnamon and ginger.

2. Add raisins and walnuts, or even a tablespoon of apple sauce. Mix in the raisins and walnuts and applesauce. Add olive oil, vanilla extract, and a pinch of salt.

4. Use a round cake pan lined with baking paper.

Bake at 350F for about 30-40 minutes.

5. The cake is cooled and sprinkled with powdered sugar.

Beetroot Cake

You can make a real, healthy, red velvet cake if you are looking for a cheaper alternative. Simply bake beets into the cake.

Servings: 4-6 dishes

Ingredients:

1/3 small beet pureed c

1 cup sugar

1/4 cup whole wheat flour.

2 tbsp. cocoa powder

One teaspoon

1/2 teaspoon baking soda

1 1/4 cup coconut milk

Vanilla extract

1/4 teaspoon of salt

Directions:

A bowl of well-mixed red beet puree and coconut oil. Add in the sugar and vanilla. Sift all the dry ingredients. 2. Fold in the cake flour mixture and then the buttermilk. 3. Add the

4. Bake in the oven for 18 to 20 minutes.

Before baking, set the oven at 350 degrees F. Bake the cake for 30-40 minutes. 5. Let the cake cool off on a wire rack for 10 minutes. Par

5. Let cool in the pan then transfer to a serving plate. Dust sugar on the cake. Serve powdered with sugar.

Simple Chocolate Cake recipe

Sometimes you want to make something sweet, but you don't want to make something that will take too long or too much work. And that's when this cake fills the gap in between because it's easy to make and tastes amazing.

Servings: 4-6 dishes

Ingredients:

1 cup all purpose flour

1 cup sugar

4 tablespoons cocoa

1 teaspoon vinegar

1 cup cold water

1 teaspoon vanilla extract

a pinch of salt

1 teaspoon baking powder

Directions:

1. Put all the ingredients in a large bowl and mix them all together.

2. While the cake is baking, set the oven temperature to 350°F, and cook the cake for 20-30 minutes.

3. Sliced with powdered sugar

Coconut Bread

If you're a coconut lover, these breads can't be beat. They are packed with coconut flavor and will give you the best of both worlds.

Servings: 4-6 dishes

Ingredients:

1/2 cup unsweetened applesauce

1/3 cup almond or soy milk

1/4 teaspoon vanilla extract

1/3 cup of all purpose flour

1 teaspoon baking powder

1/2 teaspoon baking soda.

1 teaspoon cinnamon

1 cup sugar

six tablespoons coconut oil

1 teaspoon lemon juice

1 pinch of salt

Directions:

Add applesauce, milk, and vanilla to a small bowl. Mix it well.

In a mixing bucket, combine the flour, baking powder, cinnamon, a pinch of salt and sugar in one bowl. Add the coconut flakes and mix together well. Stir in the milk mixture until all the flour is mixed in then pour the batter into a cake pan, lined with baking paper.

3. Bake at 350F for about 30-40 minutes. The edges will be lightly browned.

Ginger and Applesauce Cake

Ginger is used to flavor foods so it is wise to be careful not to overuse it. The cake is delicious and it preserves a lot of moisture from the applesauce.

Servings: 2-4 dishes

Ingredients:

2 cups whole wheat flour

1 cup sugar

2 oz candied ginger, chopped

2 tablespoons cornstarch

1 teaspoon baking soda

1 teaspoon baking powder

1 teaspoon cinnamon

You can have 2 1/2 cups applesauce.

1 teaspoon lemon juice

1 teaspoon vanilla

1 pinch of salt

2 tablespoons maple syrup

Directions:

1. Combine applesauce, lemon juice and vanilla in a bowl.

2.

The spices mix well

3. Put the liquid batter into a round cake pan with a parchment paper lining.

Bake the cake for 35-40 minutes.Insert a skewer into the center of the cake.If it comes out clean, the cake is done.If it comes out sticky, bake the cake for 10 more minutes.

Use it for cake or ice-cream.

Walnut Carrot Cake

Carrot cake with walnuts tastes great because walnuts complement the earthy carrots nicely.

Servings: 4-6 dishes

Ingredients:

10 dates, pits removed

2 cups grated carrots

1/2 cup sweetened applesauce

½ cup golden raisins

1 teaspoon cinnamon

1 teaspoon ground ginger

1/2 teaspoons ground cloves

3/4 cup whole wheat flour

1/4 cup all purpose flour

A tablespoon of baking powder

1/2 teaspoon baking soda.

½ cup walnuts, chopped

1 pinch of salt

Directions:

1. Add the dates to a food processer, then pulse until a paste forms, transfer them into a bowl and stir in the carrots, applesauce, raisins, cinnamon, ginger and salt.

2. Place the flour, baking powder and soda in a bowl or container. Add the ingredients to the bowl/container. Mix until well combined. Spoon the batter into a greased round cake pan then sprinkle the chopped walnuts on top.

Bake at 350 F for 30 to 40 minutes.

4. Let it cool, and then serve it with powdered sugar.

Strawberry Cake

Strawberries must be one of the most beloved fruits worldwide—but they also make excellent dessert desserts, like this flavorful and crumbly cake.

Servings: 4-6 dishes

Ingredients:

1/2 cup flour

2/3 cup sugar

1/3 cup * yogurt

1 teaspoon baking soda

2/3 teaspoon baking powder

1 teaspoon vanilla extract

You can start your day with 1 cup of soy milk.

2 cups fresh strawberries, coarsely chopped

2 tablespoons cornstarch

Salt

Directions:

1. In a large bowl, mix the flour, sugar, baking powder and salt as well as a small pinch of salt.

The cake batter will be stirred in the yogurt, vanilla and soy milk.

3. Fold the strawberries into the batter.

Bake the cake in a 350F oven for 40-50 minutes.

4.

When the cake is done, put it in the pan and pour honey over the top.

Banana Blueberry Cake

A banana cake is generally very moist and fragrant, but this cake is even better with the addition of blueberries. Perfectly baked, this cake is appropriate for any occasion or time of the day.

Servings: 4-6 dishes

Ingredients:

3, ripe bananas, mashed

1/2cup of soy milk

1 tablespoon vanilla extract

Agave nectar

1/4 cup sugar

2 cups whole wheat flour

1/2 teaspoon baking soda

1 1/2 teaspoon baking powder

1 cup blueberries

1/2 teaspoon of salt

Directions:

Grease a 9 inch round cake pan and set aside.

2. In a blender, blend the soy milk, the lemon juice and the nutritional yeast until smooth

3. Add the banana, agave, and sugar; mix well.

I want to make blueberry bundt cake.

The cake should be baked at 350F for 40-50 minutes, then cooled in the pan on a wire rack. It should then be transferred to a serving plate and sprinkled with powdered sugar.

Sugar cake

Cinnamon can be very strong and create a swirl effect that enhances the visual sensation of the slice.

Servings: 4-6 dishes

Ingredients:

1 cup all purpose flour

1 cup whole wheat flour

1 teaspoon baking powder

1 teaspoon baking soda

1 teaspoon cinnamon

1/2 teaspoon ground ginger

2 tablespoons flax seeds ground

4 tablespoons water

1 tablespoon of yogurt

3/4 cup orange juice

1/2 cup soy milk

1/2 cup agave syrup

1/4 cup sugar

[1 pinch of salt

Directions:

There's a bowl on the table. Add the ground flax seeds to the water in the bowl.

3. Heat a large wok or skillet over high heat. Add one tablespoon of the oil and let it get hot.

3. Add this mixture to the dry ingredients then add the flax seeds and salt.

4. Pour the batter into a cake pan.

5. Bake the cake for 40-50 minutes at 350F.

Mandarin Cake

The mandarin is similar to a common orange, but the flavor is a bit different. This cake is easy to make and perfect as a dessert, topped with coconut cream (or as an afternoon snack).

Servings: 2-4 dishes

Ingredients:

1 cup all purpose flour

3/4 cup whole wheat flour

1/2 cup brown sugar

1 teaspoon baking soda

1 cup of juice

1/4 cup coconut milk

1/2 cup

1 teaspoon of Salt

1/4 teaspoon of vanilla extract

Directions:

Add flour to a large bowl and mix with baking soda, salt, and brown sugar.

At this point, you will mix the coconut milk, oil and vanilla extract.

3.

Bake at 350 degrees for about 40 minutes, until slightly browned and fragrant.

I'm going to make you Cake

Orange and chocolate is the best flavor pair because the orange softens the flavor of the chocolate, and the chocolate enhances the natural flavor of the orange.

Servings: 4-6 dishes

Ingredients:

1 1/2 cups all purpose flour

You need 1 cup of whole wheat flour to bake a cake.

1/2 cup cornstarch

1/2 cup sugar

1 tablespoon baking soda

1/2 cup cocoa powder

3/4 cup soy yogurt

1 teaspoon cinnamon

Get 1/2 of a cup of fresh orange juice

1 Tablespoon of orange zest

1 tsp vanilla extract

Salt

Directions:

1. Mix the flour with the sugar, cornstarch, baking soda, and cocoa powder.

Place the soy yogurt, cinnamon, orange juice, vanilla extract, salt and orange zest into a bowl and mix well. Add the soy yogurt mixture into a greased round cake pan and place in the oven for 60 minutes.

Bake in a preheated oven at 350F for 30-40 minutes

Make these a few times because you'll love them.

Peach Upside-Down Cake

Upside-down cakes are very popular because the soft fruits can make the batter on the bottom of the cake silky and juicy, which makes the cake even more enjoyable.

Servings: 4-6 dishes

Ingredients:

2 1/4 cup all purpose flour

1 tablespoon baking powder

1 teaspoon cinnamon

1 teaspoon ground ginger

1/2 cup sugar

1 tsp of salt

Use 1 cup of soy milk

1 teaspoon of lemon juice

One teaspoon of lemon zest

1 pound of peaches. Cut into slices.

2 tablespoons brown sugar

Directions:

1. Combine the flour and baking powder in a bowl. Add cinnamon, ginger, sugar and salt, and stir to mix. 2. In another bowl, pour in the soy milk and lemon juice.

Add the flour. Fold in the lemon zest.

3. In a heavy skillet, pour about 3 tablespoons of oil and sprinkle brown sugar on the bottom. Arrange the peaches (you can use the peach halves instead) on top of the sugar then spoon over the batter.

4. Bake in a preheated oven at 350F for 30-40 minutes. After it is removed from the oven, let it cool in the pan for 10 minutes. Then, remove the cake from the pan and put it on a plate.

Pineapples are among the most used fruits when it comes to upside down cakes because they are juicy, but not overly juicy. When used in a cake, they bake to perfection each time. (this is a paraphrasing of the article

Servings: 4-6 dishes

Ingredients:

1 can pineapple, drained

1 cup quick oats

1/2 cup whole wheat flour

1/2 cup sugar

The mixture should be 1 teaspoon baking powder

1/4 cup flax seeds ground

2 tablespoons water

1 teaspoon cinnamon

1 teaspoon ground ginger

One pinch of salt

The amount of vanilla extract: 1 teaspoon

1/3 cup unsweetened applesauce.

3 tablespoons water

1 teaspoon lemon juice

Directions:

1. Mix the flax seeds into a bowl: 2. Add the applesauce to the flax seeds and let them soak for 5 minutes. 3. Add the vanilla, water, and lemon juice to the mixture.

Beat together the sugar, shortening, eggs, and vanilla. Combine the dry ingredients, add the milk and vanilla extract, and add in the strawberries. Pour the batter into the cake pan. Arrange the pineapple slices on the bottom of the pan

3. Pile on the batter.

Turn on the oven for 10 minutes.

Raspberry Chocolate Cake

Raspberries and chocolate

Servings: 4-6 dishes

Ingredients:

Make your pancakes with 3 cups of all purpose flour

1 cup sugar

2 teaspoons of baking soda

1/2 cup cocoa

1/4 cup coconut oil

½ cup raspberry jam

1/4 cup of applesauce, unsweetened

*2 teaspoons teaspoons white wine vinegar

2 cups water

1 1/2 tbsp of sea salt

1/2 cup raspberry jam to glaze

Directions:

1. Mix the flour, sugar, baking soda, cocoa and a pinch of salt,
2. and pour them into a bowl. Note: The phrase “a pinch of salt”

Place the cake in a preheated oven for about 35 minutes - until a skewer inserted in the cake comes out clean.

3. Cool the cake in the pan before cutting it in half. Once the cake has cooled, spread raspberry jam between the layers. This will make the cake more moist.

Cherry, Walnut and Banana Cake

As mentioned before, this banana and walnut cake has fresh spring aromas, but with a mixture of the earthiness of the banana and cherry fragrance and the freshness of the walnut and the banana, as well as the other aromas of the

Servings: 4-6 dishes

Ingredients:

3 ripe bananas, mashed

3 1 teaspoon lemon juice

cup unsweetened applesauce

1/2 cup of brown sugar

1 cup whole wheat flour

1 cup flour

1/2 cup dried cherries

1 teaspoon baking powder

1 teaspoon baking soda

1 tablespoon of walnut oil (or olive oil).

1 pinch of salt

Directions:

1. Blend the bananas with the lemon juice in a bowl.

2. Stir in the applesauce and sugar. Add the flours, baking powder, baking soda and salt. 3. Mix until a dough starts to form. 4.

Get a variety of foods to combine and fold in

4. Let the cake cool for 10 minutes in the pan, then remove and cool on a wire rack.

Serve cold with a touch of powdered sugar.

Sweet Snack Cake

This cake tastes delicious, but it's also a good choice for breakfast, snack or dessert.

Servings: 4-6 dishes

Ingredients:

1/2 teaspoon rolled

1 tablespoon flax seeds

1/2 cup whole wheat flour

1 teaspoon baking powder

1 teaspoon baking soda

1/2 tablespoon all spice powder

1/3 cup maple syrup

1/2 cup cherry juice

1 cup pitted cherries

1/2 cup applesauce

1/2 teaspoon

Directions:

To grind flax requires a lot of work. You'll have to use a food processor or blender.

In a bowl, combine the cake flour, baking powder, baking soda, and all spice powder along with a pinch of salt. Add the cherry juice, maple syrup and applesauce. Gently fold in the pitted cherries, and then distribute the mixture into a greased and floured 8-inch small cake pan.

3. Bake in a preheated oven at 350F for 40 to 50 minutes or until a skewer inserted in the center of the cake comes out clean. In making a paraphrase, you can either modify the same

Zucchini

This cake is moist and creamy and uses a healthy mix of vegetables to make it.

Despite the zucchini because it makes this cake as delicious as it is.

Servings: 4-6 dishes

Ingredients:

*2 cups whole wheat flour

1/2 cup raw sugar 1/2 cup sugar.

3/4 cup of cocoa powder

3/4 cup chickpea flour

1 teaspoon baking soda

1/2 tsp. baking powder

1 pinch of salt

3/4 cup coconut oil

1 cup water

1/2 cup grated zucchini

1 teaspoon vanilla extract

1 teaspoon cinnamon

Directions:

In a bowl, combine the flour with the brown sugar, chickpea flour, baking soda, baking powder, salt, and cinnamon.

2. Add the coconut oil, water and vanilla to the sifter. Combine the flour and baking powder. Stir in the grated zucchini. Spoon the batter into a greased bund pan and bake in a preheated oven at 350F for one hour.

3. Paraphrase uses new words and new structure to explain the ideas in the Original section and follow the following guidlines in making a paraphrase: 1- Start your first sentence at a different point from that of the original source.

Vanilla Cake Bakeswell

This is probably the most basic of fruit desserts. It can be a good base for making other desserts as it can be filled with jam or cream, frosted and transformed into a lovely celebration cake.

Servings: 4-6 dishes

Ingredients:

1/2 cup 3/4 cup brown rice flour

1/2 cup tapioca flour.

1/2 cup almond meal

1/2 cup coconut flour

1 tbsp

Baking powder (1 teaspoon)

1 Teaspoon Baking Soda (salt)

0.5 teaspoon xanthan gum

1 cup

1 cup water

1/4 cup coconut oil

1/4 cup applesauce

1 teaspoon vanilla extract1

lemon

Directions:

1. In a bowl, combine the flours with the salt, baking powder, baking soda, and xanthan gum.

In a container: Add the water to the coconut milk, coconut oil, apple sauce, vanilla extract and lemon juice. Stir with a fork to combine until smooth.

3. Grease a 9-inch cake pan or line it with baking paper then pour the batter into the pan.

At 350°F, a cake will rise and fall in approximately 1 hour. After that, it will need to be allowed to cool in the pan. The cake will continue to rise as it cools, so you may want to keep it on a platter with frosting

You will enjoy this cake so much each day that you'll want to prepare it again.

Serving: 4-6 dishes

Ingredients:

2/3 cup olive oil

1/2 cup chopped rosemary

1 pinch of salt

1/3 cup warm water

3/2 cups semolina flour

ground flax seeds, 3 tablespoons

Juice of 1 orange

1 cup sugar

Directions:

2. Add the olive oil to a frying pan. Heat it then add the rosemary for 20 minutes.

minutes and hours.

After the yeast has been added to water, wait for 10 minutes. This allows time for the yeast to be activated, or "bumped."

Mix together the orange juice, sugar, flax seeds, and semolina flour, then add a pinch of salt.

While the mixture is rising, let it "soak" for 45 minutes to 1 hour, then add the olive oil. Cover and let rise at least 2 hours.

5. Grease a 10-inch bundt cake pan with oil and flour it slightly.

Turn the oven on to 350F and bake for 40 to 60 minutes, or until risen and golden. Let it cool in the pan before serving.

Apfelkuchen

German dessert apple cake is a classic and delicious dessert. It is gluten free and made with apples, raisins, and nuts.

Servings: 4-6 dishes

Ingredients:

2 pounds apples, peeled, cored and sliced

1/2 cup solid coconut oil

1/2 cup

1/2 cup applesauce

1/4 cup soy milk

Bake at 250° F for 2 hours

1 cup whole wheat flour

1/2 teaspoon all-purpose flour

Salt

1 teaspoon cinnamon

Directions:

In a bowl, stir the coconut oil with the sugar until the mixture is creamy. Stir in the applesauce and soy milk. Add the flours, salt, and the baking powder, then spoon the batter into an 8-inch greased or lined baking pan, and spread the batter out as thinly as you can

Add an apple and sprinkle with cinnamon to top the batter.

3. Bake in a preheated oven at 350 degrees for about 20 minutes. When it's done, let it sit in the pan for a while before serving.

Blueberry Chocolate Cake

An impressive treat that includes blueberries and chocolate is created by this recipe. It's smooth and tasty, and it's worth trying!

Servings: 4-6 dishes

Ingredients:

1 cup whole wheat flour

1/4 cup all purpose flour

¼ cup cocoa powder

1 teaspoon baking powder

1/2 teaspoon baking soda.

1 teaspoon ground flax seed

3/4 cup water

1/2 cup of maple syrup

1 cup blueberries

1 pinch of salt

Directions:

Mix the flours, cocoa powder, baking powder, soda, and salt, and mix in the ground flax seeds . Paraphrase: Make a combination of flour, cocoa powder, baking powder, soda,

I poured the water into a blender with the blueberries. I pulsed the berries until they were smooth. I added the blueberries, together with the maple syrup, and stirred everything together.

Pour the batter into a greased medium-size cake pan and bake in a preheated oven at 350F for 40 – 50 minutes.

Serve sprinkled with powdered sugar.

Vegan Muffin Recipes

Vegan muffins are excellent to serve for lunch or as a part of your breakfast, as they are both delicious and healthy. Most people think that using eggs and cream improves the taste of muffins. However, using egg substitutes and butter is also an excellent way to create delicious vegan muffins.

A Blueberry Whole Wheat Muffin

These muffins are both delicious and healthy because they contain a high fiber content and are loaded with antioxidants. Strawberries can be used in place of blueberries, and raspberries in place of strawberries.

Servings: 12 muffins

Ingredients:

1 ½ cups whole wheat flour

½ cup of oat flour

2 teaspoons baking soda

1 pinch salt

½ cup agave syrup

2 tablespoons ground flax seeds

¼ cup water

½ cup coconut oil, melted.

½ cup almond milk

1 teaspoon of apple cider

blueberries with one cup fresh or frozen

Directions:

1. Mix the flour and the oat flour together. 2. Add the baking soda and salt.

2. Blend the flax seeds with water in a different bowl.

For 10 minutes, cover the seeds in the mason jars with the water and soak them overnight, as the instructions suggest. Then, add the agave syrup, coconut oil, almond milk, and cider vinegar.

4. Combine the dry ingredients that you mixed earlier, mix well, and be consistent.

Put the batter in the muffin cup and gently fold in the blueberries. Then, cook your muffins in a skillet.

Put the muffins into a preheated oven at 350°F for 20-30 minutes or until slightly golden brown and fragrant enough. Let the muffins cool in pan and serve.

The muffins in the above video are reminiscent of chocolate chip cookies. They have an even more delicious taste.

Servings: 6 muffins

Ingredients

½ cup pecans, ground

¼ cup shredded coconut

¼ cup almond butter

2 tablespoons flax seeds ground

1/4 cup coconut milk

¼ cup agave syrup

1 vanilla extract

One (teaspoon)

Directions:

1. Add the almond butter to the agave syrup, and mix to form a creamy consistency.

2. Add milk, pecans, flaxseeds and vanilla.

Spoon the chocolate chips into the muffin cups, then spoon the batter into the lined cups.

In the oven, on a rack, bake the cake. Bake for 25 minutes or until golden brown and fragrant.

Serve those muffins when they've cooled to room temperature.

Banana and Sunflower Muffins

Servings: 12 muffins

Ingredients:

Two tablespoons of ground flax seeds

¼ cup cold water

1 cup of oats

¼ cup cornstarch

½ cup almond flour

½ cup sunflower seeds, ground

1 pinch salt

1 teaspoon baking powder

½ cup sunflower oil

2 ripe bananas, mashed

Half cup of maple syrup

Directions:

Mix the ground flax seeds with cold water and let them soak in the fridge for 10 minutes.

2. Combine the mashed bananas, sunflower oil, and maple syrup.

3. Mix together the flour, cornstarch, nuts, seeds, and salt in a separate bowl.

4. Take ingredients and add them to a mixing bowl. Mix in the wet ingredients and mix well. Fill the muffin cups with

batter; bake for two hours at 350°F or until golden brown and fragrant.

Fudgy Chocolate Muffins

The special ingredients for these muffins are beets which add a fudgy earthy flavor. You can customize the recipe in any way you wish with additional fruit and/or alcohol if you wish.

Servings: 12 muffins

Ingredients:

2 tablespoons ground flax seeds

2 tablespoons water

1 large beet pureed in a blender

one-quarter cup agave syrup

½ cup maple syrup.

¼ cup coconut oil

¼ cup coconut milk;

1 pinch salt

1 teaspoon baking soda

¼ cup of cocoa powder

1 cup all-purpose flour

½ cup oat flour

Directions:

Stir the flax seeds, beets, and agave together in a bowl. Add the maple syrup, coconut oil, and coconut milk.

Stir together all the ingredients. Mix really well.

for 20 minutes or until golden brown and fragrant,

(4.)

Tropical Coconut Muffins

The fruit with coconut, pineapple, nuts, and tropical fruits in a mouth-watering combination comes together in this delicious recipe.

Servings: 12 muffins

Ingredients:

½ cup rolled oats

1 ½ cups oat flour

½ cup coconut flakes

1 teaspoon of baking powder

```js var teaspoon = 0.0393701; ```

1 pinch salt

Half a cup of soy yogurt

½ cup coconut cream
```

½ cup maple syrup.

¼ cup coconut oil

1 ripe banana, mashed

½ cup of crushed pineapple, drained.

½ cup mangos

Directions:

Add the rolled oats, oat flour, shredded coconut, baking powder, baking soda, and salt to the bowl.

A different bowl, a different blend of ingredients, and a totally different outcome.

3. Fold a pineapple and a mango into the batter and then spoon the batter into the muffin cups lining the tin.

The muffins are good after they have cooled down a bit.

Melon Muffins

Canteloupes (or melons) are delicious when eaten on their own, but they can also be used to create delicious desserts. Some of the most popular include Melon Muffins.

Servings: 12 muffins

Ingredients:

1 cup whole wheat flour

½ cup all-purpose flour

1 teaspoon baking soda

1 pinch salt

1 pinch of ground ginger

1 small melon, peeled and cubed

¼ cup of agave syrup

1 tablespoon vanilla extract

¼ cup coconut oil

Directions:

1- Use a blender to mix the melon with agave syrup. 2- Vanilla and coconut oil add flavor.

Stir the flours, baking soda, salt, and ginger into the puréed carrot until smooth.

Spread a thin layer of the batter on each muffin pan, then put pans in a hot oven. Bake at 350°F for approximately 25 minutes or until the surface is golden brown.

Multigrain Muffins

Muffins that contain a multitude of nutrients and fiber are the perfect dish for breakfast. With a cup of tea or a glass of fresh juice, your morning starts off great!

Servings: 12 muffins

Ingredients:

2 tablespoons ground flax seeds.

2 tablespoons of cold water

1 cup of almond milk

1½ cups all-purpose flour

½ cup of rolled oats

½ cup quinoa

1 teaspoon baking powder

1 pinch salt

A pinch of cinnamon powder

1½ c. purée of pumpkin

Half cup of maple syrup.

¼ cup pumpkin seeds

½ cup sunflower seeds

2 cups of unsalted and organic, unsmoked, bacon ends

Directions:

Put the ground flax seeds in a bowl and add the cold water.

2. After soaking for 5 minutes, stir in the almond milk, vinegar, pumpkin purée, and maple syrup.

3. Add the flour, oats, quinoa, baking powder, salt, and cinnamon powder.

Add pumpkin seeds, sunflower seeds, and poppy seeds.

Remove the muffins from the pan for storage, at least an hour after baking.

76

Almond Cranberry Muffins

It's always a good time to start your day with a warm muffin that's just right. This muffin is soft and moist on the inside and crunchy on the outside. This is an excerpt of an in-

Servings: 12 muffins

Ingredients:

2 cups rolled oats

1 ripe banana, mashed.

1 cup pumpkin purée

cup almond butter

¼ cup almond milk

½ cup

½ cup dried cranberries, chopped.

.25 teaspoon cinnamon

1 pinch salt

to ½ tsp Use a combination of the above paraphrases. A

½ cup sliced almonds for topping

Directions:

1. Add the mashed banana, puréed pumpkin, almond butter, milk, and maple syrup to a mixing bowl. 2. Combine 3. Mix

4. Combine oats, cranberries, milk, baking soda, cream of tartar and cinnamon in a large bowl.

5. The cookies should be baked for 25 to 30 minutes or until they are completely crispy and golden brown.

Serve the muffins when they are cool.

Ginger and Banana Muffins

Ginger is used with bananas, but this combination is particularly special. The aroma from the ginger is mild and lovely, with the softness of the banana muffins.

Servings: 12 muffins

Ingredients:

2/4 cups all-purpose flour

1 teaspoon baking soda

Baking powder is 1 teaspoon

1 pinch salt

1 teaspoon ground ginger

* cup coconut oil*

½ cup applesauce

2 ripe bananas, mashed

cup coconut milk

Directions:

1. Combine the flour, baking soda, baking powder, and salt. Add ginger, organic applesauce, bananas, and coconut milk.
2. Add the pineapple. Paraphrase: The

2. Spoon the batter, as directed in step 1 Fry the buns.

Leave the muffins to cool completely before serving or storing

Plum Muffins

Pears are so underrated - they are so delicious and delicious; but they are also underrated.

Servings: 12 muffins

Ingredients:

1+ ¾ cups oat flour.

1 pinch salt

1teaspoon baking soda.

Half a teaspoon of cinnamon powder

1 cup agave syrup

1 cup silken tofu

1 teaspoon of vanilla

1/4 cup coconut oil, melted.

2 tablespoons ground flax seeds

8 plums, pitted and diced

Directions:

1. Mix the oat flour with the salt, baking soda and cinnamon and set aside.

Two. Combine silken tofu with agave syrup, vanilla, coconut oil, and flax seeds to form a smooth, creamy mixture.

3. Make a paste of these ingredients

4. Plums folded with muffin batter and baked to golden brown.

Blackberry Muffins **NOTE: The paragraph should be in the same font size, same format,

To retain the light, airy texture of muffins, I chose cornstarch as the binding agent. I also added in cranberries to add a bit of sweetness and to help infuse the muffins with the cranberry taste.

Servings: 12 muffins

Ingredients:

1 cup cornstarch

1/2 cup all-purpose flour

1 teaspoon baking powder.

1 pinch of cinnamon powder

1 pinch salt

¾ cup applesauce

1/2 cup coconut milk

½ cup agave syrup

1 teaspoon of vanilla extract

1 cup blackberries

Directions:

Combine the flours with the baking powder and cinnamon. Add the applesauce, coconut milk, agave syrup, and vanilla.

2. You want to fold the fruit into your muffins before spooning the batter on the pan.

Bake in a preheated oven at 350°F for about 20-30 minutes.

It's important to check the muffins at the end of the cooking time.

5. If the muffins are a few minutes away from being finished, and there are a few crumbs in the oven, then the muffins need a few more minutes baking.

Allow the muffins to cool in the pan after they're done cooking.

Sweet potato ginger muffins

I'm sure you've had pumpkin muffins before, but this is also true of sweet potatoes. Sweet potato provides a similar consistency, so why not use it in baking? These final muffins are sweet and fragrant, yet they are also rich and filling.

Servings: 12 muffins

Ingredients:

2 cups whole wheat flour

1 teaspoon baking soda

1 pinch salt

1 teaspoon cinnamon powder

½ teaspoon ground cloves

1 teaspoon grated ginger

1 tablespoon

½ cup coconut oil

2 tablespoons ground flax seeds

A ½ cup of almond milk

¾ cup maple syrup

1 large sweet potato, baked and mashed

1 sweet potato, grated

½ cup pecans, chopped

Directions:

1. In a bowl, combine the flour with the baking soda, salt, cinnamon, and ground cloves. Set aside.

In a medium bowl, combine the coconut oil, grated ginger, vanilla, milk, and maple syrup.

A: 3. B: Scoop the dry, seasoned mix into a large bowl and mix in the grated sweet potato and chopped pecans.

Spoon your batter into lined muffin cups.

5. Prepare a loaf of bread in a preheated oven at 350°F for 20-25 minutes or until golden brown and fragrant. Allow the loaf to cool in the pan before slicing.

Quinoa Raspberry Muffins

Quinoa, also known as a grain that can be mistaken for couscous, is the super food of the century. Aside from using it in foods, it can also be added to desserts to boost the nutritional content.

Servings: 12 muffins

Ingredients:

A half cup of quinoa, toasted

¼ cup

2 cups all-purpose flour.

½ cup cornstarch

1¼ teaspoons...

1 pinch salt

½ cup agave syrup

2 tablespoons of orange zest

1 cup of almond milk

(cup)

¼ cup coconut oil, melted

[1 teaspoon of vanilla extract]

1 and 1/2 cup fresh raspberries

Directions:

Cook the quinoa in a saucepan over medium heat for a few minutes and stir in the orange juice. Let it cool and put the quinoa in a bowl.

2. Pour in your agave, almond milk, orange juice, coconut oil, vanilla, the other half cup of orange juice, and stir with a wooden spoon.

4. Add the milk.

4. Add the raspberries in last.

The batter should be divided among your muffin cups and you should bake them in a preheated oven at 350°F for 20-30 minutes or until golden brown and well risen.

Allow the muffins to cool in the pan and then serve.

Applesauce Cardamom Muffins

The applesauce pairs well with the ground cardamom used in this muffin. You could also add fresh apple slices, if you want to enhance the flavor.

Servings: 12 muffins

Ingredients:

1 cup of coconut milk

1 cup applesauce

¼ cup agave syrup.

1 tsp lemon juice

2 tablespoons of ground flax seeds

1 pinch salt

1 tablespoon baking soda.

1 teaspoon ground ginger

1/2 teaspoon

¾ cups all-purpose flour

½ cup almond flour

Directions:

1. Cook the coconut milk and applesauce together and then add the agave syrup and lemon juice

Mix in the flours, ground ginger, and cardamom.

To make these muffins, first spoon the batter into a muffin pan. Then place these muffins in a preheated oven at 350 degrees F for about 30 minutes. The muffin tops are golden brown and fragrant. They are ready to serve once

Goji berries give muffins a great flavor and antioxidant content, making them a healthy snack. These muffins are moist and dense, almost fudgy-like in consistency and are absolutely delicious.

Servings: 12 muffins

Ingredients:

1/2 cup whole wheat flour

1 teaspoon baking soda

1 teacup baking powder

1 teaspoon cinnamon powder

1 pinch salt

2 Tbsp cocoa powder

1 cup almond milk

1 teaspoon of vanilla extract

¼ cup agave syrup

¼ cup chopped Goji berries

Directions:

1.

Take the following ingredients into a bowl: sugar, whole wheat flour, cocoa powder, baking soda, baking powder, cinnamon, salt.

2. Stir in the coconut oil, vanilla extract, almond milk and agave syrup.

Three. Add ghee

In your muffin pan, place the muffin batter so that each muffin cup is filled almost to the top. Bake the muffins in a preheated oven for 20 to 30 minutes, or until they are fragrant and golden brown.

Serve these delicious muffins hot from the oven. Once they are cool, they are ready to be eaten.

Walnut and Chia Muffins

These muffins are a great source of fiber and that makes them perfect for breakfast. Have them along with some orange juice, and you're set to enjoy a great day ahead.

Servings: 12 muffins

Ingredients:

1 ½ cups of almond milk

½ cup applesauce

1 teaspoon apple cider vinegar

1 cup all-purpose flour

½ cup whole wheat flour

1. teaspoon of baking soda

2 tablespoons chia seeds

1/2 teaspoon cinnamon powder"

1/3 cup walnuts, chopped

1 pinch salt

Directions:

1. Boil the water and mix the almond milk with the vinegar and applesauce.

Add the flours to the mixing bowl, followed by the baking soda, chia seeds, cinnamon powder, and salt.

3 cups of walnuts and spoon the batter into muffin cups.

When they're ready, bake the muffins in a preheated oven. They should be fragrant and golden brown.

Make sure they've cooled first

Pumpkin Millet Muffins

It's not advisable to make muffins for humans when other kinds of ingredients are used. However, millet flour is a good option in baking, as it not only brings taste and texture to the muffin, but also brings fiber and other nutrients in it.

Servings: 16 muffins

Ingredients:

2 tablespoons of ground flax seeds

4 tablespoons water

½ cup coconut oil

Agave syrup

1. cup coconut milk.

1 (cup) ¾ cup pumpkin purée

½ cup rolled oats

1 cup millet

1½ cups whole wheat flour

1 tsp of baking soda

1 tablespoon baking powder

1 pinch salt

1 teaspoon of cinnamon

Directions:

Combine the ground flax seeds with 6-8 oz of water in a food processor, but don't process in the food processor.

After combining the flour mixture and coconut oil, add the liquid and mix well. Then combine the remaining ingredients and mix well.

4. In this case, mix it well, and transfer the batter to muffin cups.

It's better served when hot.

Gluten-Free Cupcakes

These muffins are ideal if you have a gluten allergy or intolerance, because they are made without gluten. This recipe doesn't sacrifice on taste, but instead uses healthy and nutritious ingredients to create moist, dense, and delicious muffins that are great for helping you with your sweet cravings.

Servings: 12 muffins

Ingredients:

2 cups ground flax seeds

4 tablespoons cold water, 4 tablespoons cold water

To get the full effect, eat 1½ cups of pumpkin on a daily basis

¼ cup agave syrup

A ¼ cup of sunflower oil.

1 teaspoon vanilla extract

¾ cup sorghum flour

1 cup rice flour

½ cup oats

1/2 cup arrowroot powder

1 teaspoon baking soda # Borrowing Words From Other Languages

1 pinch salt

2 teaspoon ground cardamom

½ teaspoon ground cloves

¼ teaspoon cinnamon powder

Directions:

Add the vanilla, oil, and agave. Mix the flax seeds with the cold water. Then add the pumpkin purée, agave syrup, vanilla, and oil.

2. Combine all the dry ingredients in a large mixing bowl. Add the wet ingredients in a different bowl and mix by hand until the mixture is smooth and the dry ingredients are distributed

3. Before you take your muffin out of the oven, make sure to put the muffin papers on top of the muffins just in case the muffins overflow.

4. Preheat the oven to 350°F and bake the muffins for 20-30 minutes. They should rise and become golden brown.

Take the muffins out of the oven, and allow them to cool in the pan.

Peanut Butter Muffins

Peanut butter is a simple recipe that takes just minutes to bake. However, the taste permeates the muffins so they are very sweet and yummy.

Servings: 10-12 muffins

Ingredients:

1½ cups of all-purpose flour

1 cup oats

¼ teaspoon

1 pinch salt

1 pinch nutmeg

½ cup agave syrup

1/2-cup peanut butter

1 (1) cup almond milk

Directions:

Add 1 tsp. of peanut butter to your agave syrup.

2. Add the almond milk to a large bowl and stir in the flour, oats, cocoa powder, salt, and nutmeg until well combined.

3. Fill the muffin cups with the batter, then put the papers in the pan.

4.

Remove the muffins from the oven and allow them to cool.

Vanilla Muffins

These muffins demonstrate that it is possible to use any type of nut and the flavor still stands out in each one. It is well known that the most used aroma is vanilla but it has a lot to offer.

Servings: 16 muffins

Ingredients:

2½ cups all-purpose flour

A teaspoon of baking soda

1 teaspoon

1 pinch salt

½ cup agave syrup

2 cups almond milk.

½ cup water

1 teaspoon vinegar

1/2 teaspoon vanilla extract

¼ cup coconut oil

1 vanilla pod, split lengthwise

Directions:

1. Put the flour, baking soda, baking powder, and salt in a mixing bowl; set aside. 2. Put the butter and shortening in another mixing bowl.

2. In another bowl, combine the coconut milk, agave syrup, water, vinegar, vanilla, and the vanilla seeds.

The dry ingredients are first poured on the wet ingredients and mixed well

Spread the batter into all the muffin cups and bake for approximately 20 minutes.

For 20-30 minutes until the muffins turn slightly golden brown and fragrant.

Let the muffins cool before serving.

Vegan Cookies

The lovely aroma of fresh fruit, the beautiful flavors of food, and the soothing sounds of nature can make a moment so happy. I have found that I don't find the same joy when I am vegan. However, with some modifications to favorite recipes, vegans can enjoy the crunchy and delicious taste of cookies.

Most people are surprised at how little work it takes to make cookies without eggs or milk. After several attempts, a person finds that egg mixtures can be substituted for milk, and that soy milk is preferable to cow's milk.

In this chapter there are 32 original recipes for very healthy cookies. I can promise you that when you start making them, you will be glad that you chose to stay longer and that you're taking the time to prepare such delicious, healthy cookies.

Simple Chocolate Cookies

Chocolate cookies

Yields: 2 dozen

Ingredients:

1 cup whole wheat bread flour

1 cup golden raisins

1/2 cup rolled oats

½ cup brown sugar

2 tablespoons cocoa powder.

4 tablespoons coconut oil

1/4 cup water

1 tsp of Salt

Directions:

1. Add the chocolate chips, granola, oatmeal, granulated sugar, cocoa powder and oil to a bowl.

If the dough is too dry, add water and mix with a spoon until smooth.

Wet your hands and form small dough balls.

4. Arrange the lemons in a baking pan lined with aluminum foil.

5- Let the tray cool in the oven.

Don't forget to eat breakfast.

What are some banana cookies recipes?

Servings: 4-6 dozen

Ingredients:

2/3 cup rolled oats

2 ripe bananas, mashed

1/4 cup of coconut oil

4 tablespoons agave syrup

1 cup mixed dried

2/3 cup dark chocolate chip cookies

2/3 cup almonds sliced

2 tablespoons flax seeds in your bread

4 tablespoons water

1 tablespoon baking soda

1 pinch of salt

Directions:

1. Create a nut milk by mixing ground flax seeds with water, and set aside.

I placed bananas, chocolate chips, coconut oil and agave syrup in a bowl.

Add the dry ingredients, including the oats, dried fruits, nuts, seeds, and salt. Stir until very well combined.

4. Drop spoonfuls of dough into a pan.

Bake cookies in 10 minutes and they are ready to eat.

Chocolate Chip Cookies

A piece of chocolate and some cookies are not enough to satisfy a snack or a meal. They can make a real treat to enjoy in your leisure times.

Yields: 2 dozen

Ingredients:

One tablespoon of this has five grams of fat.

2/3 cup sugar

1 teaspoon vanilla extract

2 tablespoons of almond or coconut milk

1 cup whole wheat flour

1/2 cup almond meal

1 teaspoon baking powder.

1/2 tablespoon baking soda

3/4 cup of dark chocolate chips

3/4 cup chopped walnuts

You won't gain any benefits if you don't use salt.

Directions:

In the mixer, combine the butter and sugar and whip until smooth and creamy. Add vanilla almond milk and mix well.

2. Mix the flour, almond meal, baking soda, baking powder and a salt. Pour the cookie dough into the pan, and press the dough into the pan to form an even layer. Sprinkle the dough with the chocolate chips, and stick your thumbs

3.

4. Baked the cookies at 350F for 10-15 minutes.

7.

Oatmeal and chocolate chip cookies.

A chocolate and oatmeal cookie is a healthy way to indulge your taste in chocolate.

Yields: 3 dozen

Ingredients:

Cup of almond butter

2/3 cup sugar

2 tablespoons flaxseeds ground

4 tablespoons water

1 teaspoon baking powder

1/2 teaspoon baking soda

1/2 teaspoon vanilla extract

2/3 cup white all purpose flour

1/2 cup rolled oats

1/2 cup chocolate chips topped with icing or icing with

Use a pinch of salt.

Directions:

1. In a small bowl, pour the ground flax seeds into a bowl of water. Let it soak for fifteen minutes.

In a bowl, combine the sugar and the butter until creamy.

Make a well in the middle and add the flax eggs, vanilla, flour, oats, baking soda and baking powder, along with a pinch of salt. Mix well.

Bake the cake by using the recipe to fold in the chocolate chips, then drop spoonfuls of batter in the baking pans. Bake in a preheated oven at 350F for 15-20 minutes.

Keep it in an airtight container for up to 2 weeks.

Peanut Butter Cookies

Most people like peanut butter, but many don't use it in desserts due to its natural flavor, but I think these cookies enhance the taste of peanut butter.

Yields: 3 dozen

Ingredients:

1/2 cup peanut butter

1/2 cup applesauce

1 cup of peanuts

1/2 cup whole wheat flour

2 tablespoons flax seeds, ground

4 tablespoons water

1/2 cup sugar

1 teaspoon

1 teaspoon baking powder

1/4 teaspoon baking soda

Directions:

1. Use a small bowl or cup to soak flax seeds in water.

In a bowl, stir the peanut butter, applesauce, flax seed mixture, and a pinch of salt.

Mix

5. Mix in the flours and baking powder and soda.

4. Take spoonfuls of batter and form small balls onto greased baking trays lined with baking paper. Using a fork, press each

ball a bit to make a mark from the spoon, then place them on the baking trays.

5. Bake in a preheated oven at 350 for 15 to 17 minutes, or until fragrant. Store in an airtight container for one to two weeks.

Banana Maple Oatmeal Cookies

On a warm summer day, the combination of banana, maple syrup and oatmeal is a great breakfast idea but you can also enjoy this tasty recipe in the afternoon when you have time to get a snack.

Yields: 3 dozen

Ingredients:

1/4 cup rolled oats b

1 cup whole wheat flour

1 teaspoon baking soda

1/4 teaspoon baking powder

1 teaspoon cinnamon

1/4 teaspoon flax seeds

2 tablespoons water

1/2 cup maple syrup

1 ripe banana, mashed

1/2 cup golden raisins

1 teaspoon

1 pinch of salt

Directions:

1. Start by grinding flax seeds in a high speed blender until it has been fully ground.

2. 1\. [1. Add the oats, flour, baking powder and cinnamon, 1 pinch of salt and cinnamon, and the raisins to a large bowl; mix well.] 2. In another bowl, mix

Stir a 1 cup of flaxseed and a mashed banana, lemon, and a teaspoon of maple syrup in a large bowl, until well blended. Next, drop the batter into a cooking pan lined with parchment paper. 2.

When the cookies were baked, they were a light golden brown. They were baked in a preheated oven at 375F for 10-12 minutes. They were baked for 10 minutes. They were baked for 11 minutes. You can find the actual video

Tofu Pumpkin Cookies

Tofu is a bit too mild and doesn't have a strong, distinctive taste. Its saltiness works well to complement pumpkin.

Yields: 3 dozen

Ingredients:

1/3 cup whole wheat flour

3/4 cup all-purpose flour

1/2 cup rolled oats

1 teaspoon baking soda

1 teaspoon cinnamon

1/2 teaspoon ground ginger

1

2/3 cup

1 C. pumpkin puree

2.3 oz firm tofu, well crumbled

1 teaspoon of vanilla extract

Directions:

In a bowl, mix the flours, oats, baking soda, ginger, cinnamon, nutmeg, and a bit of salt.

2. Put the agave syrup, pumpkin puree, crumbled tofu, and vanilla extract in the blender and mix until well blended.

2. Scoop the batter into the small cups, and bake for 15-20 minutes.

4. After you've done this, let them cool in the pan and then transfer them into an airtight container to store in the refrigerator until serving.

CPSIA information can be obtained
at www.ICGtesting.com
Printed in the USA
LVHW060215160722
723616LV00015B/800

9 781804 768617